Amazing Dash Diet Breakfast Recipes for Busy People

A Complete List of Delicious Recipes to Start Your Day with Taste

Maya Wilson

Table of contents

Poached Eggs with Hollandaise and Bacon

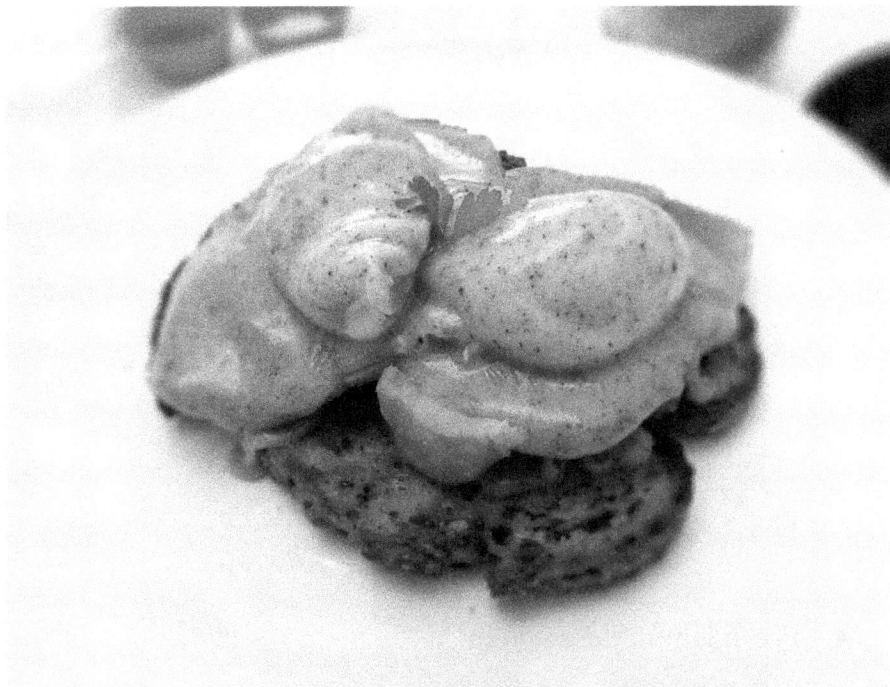

With this slimmed-down hollandaise, it is easy to enjoy a version of eggs Benedict that is SmartPoints-friendly. The sauce also makes an excellent combination with steamed asparagus or grilled salmon fillets.

Smart Points value: Green plan – 7SP, Blue plan – 5SP, Purple plan – 5SP

Total Time: 26 min, Prep time: 12 min, Cooking time: 14 min, Serves: 4

Nutritional value: Calories – 677.3, Carbs – 29.2g, Fat – 47.8g, Protein - 31.4g

Ingredients

- Plain fat-free yogurt - ¼ cup(s)

- Reduced-calorie mayonnaise - ¼ cup(s)

- Dijon Mustard - 1 tsp

- Uncooked Canadian bacon - 4 slice(s)

- Lemon zest - ½ tsp

- Egg(s) - 4 item(s), large

- Fresh lemon juice - 1 tsp

- Fresh tomato(es) - 4 slice(s), thick

- Unsalted butter - 2 tsp, softened

- Chives - 2 Tbsp, chopped fresh (optional)

- English muffin - 2 item(s), multigrain or whole wheat variety, split and toasted

- White wine vinegar - 1 Tbsp

Instructions

1. To prepare the sauce, get a small microwavable bowl and whisk yogurt, mayonnaise, mustard, and lemon zest and juice together in the bowl.

2. Set the microwave to High, and allow the mixture to heat up for about 30 seconds. Remove the bowl from the microwave carefully using your mitts.

3. Scoop a tablespoon of butter and stir it in until melted. Cover the bowl to keep your sauce warm.

4. Poach eggs by filling a large, deep skillet with water and allow to boil; add vinegar.

5. Reduce the heat to a bare simmer. Carefully break the eggs into a custard cup, one at a time, and slip into the hot water.

6. Cook the eggs until the whites are firm, but the yolks are still soft. This process should take about 5 minutes.

7. Transfer the eggs, one at a time, with a slotted spoon to a paper towel-lined plate to drain. Cover the plate to keep the eggs warm.

8. Wipe the skillet dry with a paper towel.

9. Add four slices of Canadian bacon and cook over medium-high heat until they brown in spots, about 60 seconds per side.

10. Place one half each of the English muffins on four plates.

11. Top each with one slice of bacon, one slice of tomato, one poached egg, and about two tablespoons sauce. Speckle with chives, if using.

Note: You can keep the hollandaise sauce warm for up to 40 minutes before serving.

Nut-crusted Mahi-mahi

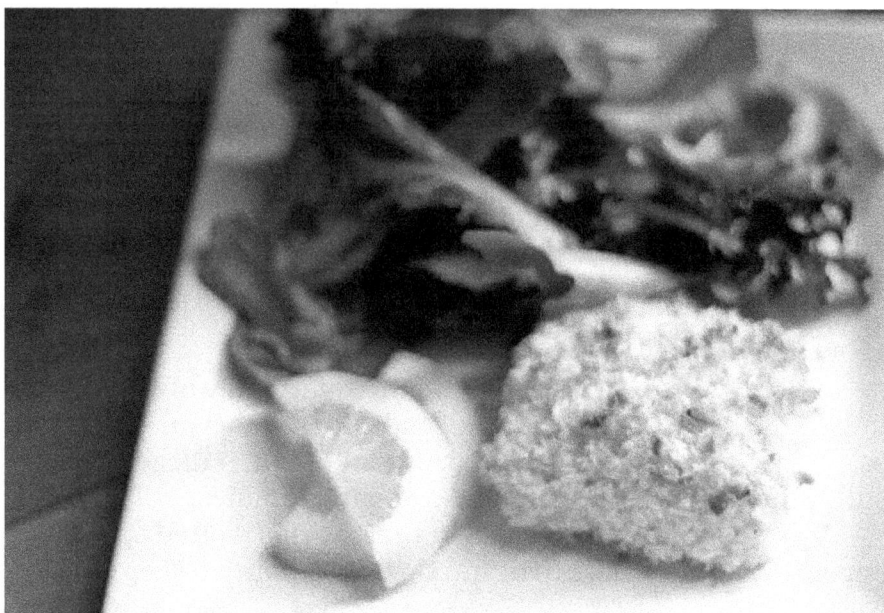

This recipe sounds fantastic and preparing it is super easy; it only takes about 20 minutes. It works well with just about any thin fish fillet and any kind of nuts. I will like you to add macadamia nuts here for their rich and buttery flavor and because they pair well together with the panko. Also, the mahi-mahi is firm enough to withstand the dredging and roasting. You are free to experiment with whatever you have in your fridge.

SmartPoints value: Green plan - 3SP, Blue plan - 2SP, Purple plan - 2SP Total Time: 20 min, Prep time: 8 min, Cooking time: 12 min, Serves: 4 Nutritional value: Calories - 234.1, Carbs - 13.9g, Fat - 9.8g, Protein - 24.7g
Ingredients

- Cooking spray - 2 spray(s)

- Egg white(s) (whipped) - 1 large

- Macadamia nuts (dry roasted, salted) - 3 Tbsp, chopped

- Mahi-mahi fillet(s) (uncooked) - 1 pound(s), no skin

- Parsley (fresh) - 2 Tbsp, or cilantro (fresh, minced)

- Plain breadcrumbs (dried) - ¼ cup(s), panko (Japanese variety)
- Table salt - ¾ tsp (divided)

Instructions

1.   Prepare the oven by preheating to 450°F. Coat a baking pan with cooking spray and place the container in the oven to heat.
2.   Place some nuts, parsley (or cilantro), panko, and 1/4 tsp of salt in a small blender, then blend all together.
3.   Pour the crumbs into a shallow bowl or plate and set the plate aside.
4.   With the fish placed on a plate, rub 1/2 teaspoon of salt all over it.

5.   Dip the fish into the egg white and turn it to coat. After that, dip the fish into the blended nut mixture and turn to coat.
6.   Remove the pan from the oven and place the coated fish on it.

7.   Roast the fish until the center of the fish is no longer translucent; about 10 to 12 minutes. Serve it immediately once it is ready.

Note: If you desire it, you can garnish with salt and pepper, but that could affect the Smart Points value.

Pan-Fried Flounder

You can serve this dish with homemade fries, or you can add freshly sliced tomatoes alongside. Bear in mind that the cooking time will be different depending on the size of your fillets.

SmartPoints value: Green plan - 4SP, Blue plan - 3SP, Purple plan - 3SP Total Time: 20 min, Prep time: 14 min, Cooking time: 6 min, Serves: 4 Nutritional value: Calories - 441.2, Carbs - 14.8g, Fat - 30.3g, Protein - 8.3g Ingredients

- Black pepper (freshly ground) - ½ tsp (or to taste)

- Cornmeal (yellow) - ¼ cup(s)

- Dijon mustard - 1 Tbsp

- Egg white(s) (whipped) - 1 large

- Lemon(s) - ½ medium, cut into four wedges

- Olive oil cooking spray - 2 spray(s)

- Olive oil - 1 Tbsp

- Parmesan cheese (grated) - 2 Tbsp

- Thyme (fresh) - 1 Tbsp, or 1 tsp dried thyme

- Table salt - ½ tsp (or to taste)

- Uncooked flounder fillet(s) - 1 pound(s)

Instructions

1.   Wash the fish with clean water and pat it dry. Place the fish on a plate and sprinkle both sides of fish with mustard, then dip it into the egg white and set aside.
2.   Mix cornmeal, thyme, Parmesan cheese, salt, and pepper in a medium bowl, then dust the fish with cornmeal-mixture. Ensure that to cover both sides.
3.   Get a large oven-proof skillet and coat it with cooking spray, then set it over medium to medium-high heat. Apply heat to the oil until it starts shimmering.
4.   Add the fish to the skillet and cook for 2 to 3 minutes on one side, then flip the fish and cook until it is ready on the other side; about 2 to 3 minutes.
5.   Serve the fish with your lemon wedges.

Blueberry-Almond Oatmeal

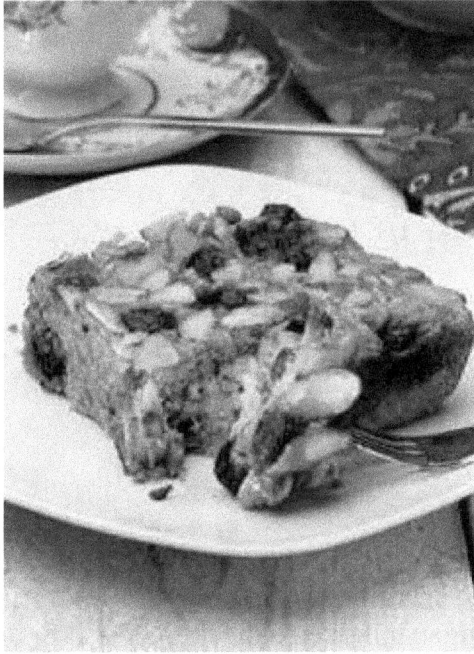

SmartPoints value: Green plan - 3SP, Blue plan - 3SP, Purple plan - 1SP Total time: 10 min, Prep time: 2 min, Cooking time: 5 min, Serves: 1 Nutritional value: Calories - 340, Carbs - 54g Fat - 8g, Protein - 16g
Ingredients

- Blueberries (fresh) - ¼ cup(s)

- Almond milk (unsweetened) - 2 Tbsp

- Slivered almonds - 2 tsp (toasted)

- Old-fashioned rolled oats (such as Quaker Oats) - 1 cup

- Milk - 1 cup

- Water - 1 cup

- Kosher salt - 1/8 tsp

- Ground cinnamon - 1/2 tsp

- Honey - 1 tsp

Instructions

1.   To prepare oatmeal, combine oats, water, milk, salt, and cinnamon in a medium-sized saucepan. Get it to boil on medium-high heat, and reduce heat to low; about 4-5 min.
2.   Simmer it uncovered until it thickens, occasionally stirring. Remove it from the heat and allow to cool slightly.
3.   Stir blueberries and milk into the oatmeal, then sprinkle it with almonds and cinnamon. Add artificial sweetener to taste if you desire.

Toasted Blueberry Muffin with Warm Citrus Compote

SmartPoints value: Green plan - 4SP, Blue plan - 4SP, Purple plan - 4SP Total Time: 20 min, Prep time: 10 min, Cooking time: 10 min, Serves: 6 Nutritional value: Calories - 231, Carbs - 36.3g Fat - 7.7g, Protein - 5.2g

Ingredients

- Brown sugar (Splenda) blend - 1 tsp

- Cornstarch - 1 Tbsp

- Water - 2 Tbsp

- Orange juice (fresh) - ½ cup(s)

- Orange sections - 1 cup(s), divided

- Vanilla extract - ⅛ teaspoon

- Lemon zest - ⅛ teaspoon

- Lime zest - ⅛ teaspoon

- WW Blueberry muffin - 3 item(s)

Instructions

1.   Prepare the oven by preheating to 350°F.

2.   Whisk cornstarch, brown sugar, and water together in a medium-sized saucepan.

3.   Whip the mixture in orange juice. While whipping constantly, bring the mixture to a boil over medium heat; about 2 minutes. The mixture will thicken rapidly, so make sure to whisk continuously to prevent lumps.

4.   Whisk the thick mixture in half cup of orange segments and continue to simmer over medium-low heat for another 6 to 8 minutes, stirring it regularly. The orange sections should break down, and the sauce should become thick, but it should not stiffen up.

5.   Drop the thick sauce from the heat and stir in vanilla extract, lemon zest, and lime zest. Allow it to cool off for about 10 minutes.

6.   While the sauce is getting cooled, cut each muffin in half and toast them in the oven lightly on both sides.

7.   Serve each person half a muffin topped with two tablespoons of compote. Garnish them with the remaining half cup of orange segments.

Notes: You can also use leftover compote as a delicious breakfast marmalade. Spread it on whole-wheat toast, apple slices, or stir it into fat-free plain yogurt. Preserve the leftover compote in an airtight container inside a refrigerator for up to 3 days.

Cuban Black Beans and Rice

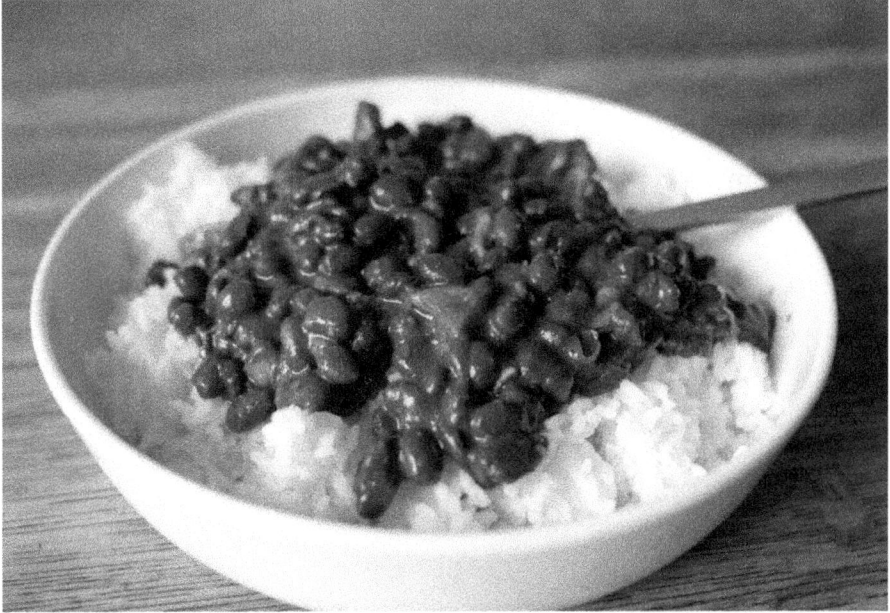

SmartPoints value: Green plan - 7SP, Blue plan - 4SP, Purple plan - 4SP

Total Time: 35 min, Prep time: 10 min, Cooking time: 25 min, Serves: 6

Nutritional value: Calories - 333.5, Carbs - 54.8g Fat - 5.1g, Protein - 16.1g
Ingredients

- Water - 2½ cup(s), divided

- Uncooked white rice (long grain-variety) - 1 cup(s)

- Olive oil - 2 tsp

- Banana pepper(s) - 1 medium

- Black beans (canned) - 31 oz, two 15.5 oz cans (undrained)

- Cilantro (fresh, chopped, divided) - ⅔ cup(s)

- Minced garlic - 1½ Tbsp
- Ground cumin - 1 tsp

- Uncooked red onion(s) (chopped) - 1¾ cup(s)

- Oregano (dried) - 1 tsp

- Table salt - 1 tsp (or to taste)

- Red wine vinegar - 1 Tbsp

- Lime(s) (fresh) - 1 medium, cut into six wedges

Instructions

1.   Bring two cups of water to a boil in a small saucepan and add the rice, then cook as package directs.

2.   Heat some oil in a large nonstick skillet over medium-high heat.

3. Add a cup of chopped onions and all of the pepper, then cook, occasionally stirring, until it is tender; about 7 minutes.

4. Toss in garlic, cumin, and oregano, then cook, stirring until fragrant; about 30 seconds.

5. Stir in the beans and their liquid, the remaining half cup of water and salt, then bring to a simmer.

6. Reduce the heat to low and simmer for the flavors to blend in about 5 minutes.

7. Remove the dish from heat, then stir in vinegar and 1/3 cup of cilantro.

8. To serve, use a spoon to put beans over rice and sprinkle it with 1/4 cup of the remaining onion and 1/3 cup of the remaining cilantro, then squeeze fresh lime juice over the top.

Note: If you desire, sprinkle the dish with salt before serving.

Spaghetti Squash With Fresh Tomato-Basil Sauce

SmartPoints value: Green plan - 2SP, Blue plan - 2SP, Purple plan - 2SP

Total time: 30 min, Prep time: 15 min, Cooking time: 15 min, Serves: 4

Nutritional value: Calories - 216.2, Carbs - 14.2g Fat - 17.2g, Protein - 5.0g

Enjoy this recipe with its taste of summer. Ensure to cook it with very ripe tomatoes and fresh basil to get the best flavour.

Ingredients

- Tomato(es) (fresh) - 2¼ pound(s)

- Olive oil (extra virgin) - 2 Tbsp

- Minced garlic - 1¼ tsp, finely minced

- Basil (fresh, sliced) - ½ cup(s)

- Kosher salt - ½ tsp (or to taste)
- Black pepper (freshly ground) - ¼ tsp (or to taste)

- Spaghetti squash (uncooked) - 2½ pound(s)

Instructions

1.   Toss tomatoes, oil, garlic, basil, salt and pepper together in a large bowl and let it stand, occasionally tossing, until the tomatoes release their juices and the mixture is quite juicy; about 10 to 15 minutes.

2.   Cut the spaghetti squash in half and scoop out the seeds, then place the squash in a covered microwave-safe container.
3.   Cook the spaghetti squash on high power until strands of squash separate when you scrape the flesh with a fork; about 15 minutes. Alternatively, you can also roast the squash for about 20 minutes in the oven.
4.   Scrape the spaghetti squash from the peel with a fork to form strands and add it to the bowl with tomatoes and toss to coat.
5.   Notes: It would be delicious to add chunks of fresh mozzarella or freshly grated Parmesan cheese to this meal. However, it might affect the Smart Points value.

Barley, Grape Tomato And Arugula Sauté

SmartPoints value: Green plan - 3SP, Blue plan - 3SP, Purple plan - 1SP

Total time: 50 min, Prep time: 10 min, Cooking time: 40 min, Serves: 4

Nutritional value: Calories - 82.8, Carbs - 4.8g Fat - 7.2g, Protein - 1.2g

This grain and vegetable side dish is colourful and sweet with a peppery bite.

Toss in some yellow grape tomatoes to add even more colour.

Ingredients

- Water - 1¼ cup(s)

- Table salt - ¾ tsp, divided

- Pearl barley (uncooked) - ½ cup(s)

- Olive oil (extra-virgin) - 1½ tsp, divided
- Tomatoes (grape) - 1½ cup(s), halved

- Minced garlic - 1½ tsp

- Black pepper (freshly ground) - ¼ tsp
- Arugula (baby leaves) - 3 cup(s)

- Lemon zest (finely grated) - ¼ tsp (or to taste)

Instructions

1.   Stir half tsp of salt into a small saucepan of water and bring it to a boil. Add barley to it and cover; reduce the heat to low and cook until the water is absorbed and the barley is tender but still has a nice bite to it; about 30-35 minutes. Remove the saucepan from the heat and set it aside.

2.   Apply heat to one teaspoon of oil in a medium nonstick skillet over medium-high heat. Add the tomatoes and garlic, then sauté it until the tomatoes start to soften and release their juices; about 1-2 minutes.

3.   Put in more barley, the remaining one-quarter teaspoon of salt and

pepper, and reduce the heat to medium and cook, stirring it until the tomatoes soften further and the grain absorbs tomato liquid; about 2-3 minutes.

4.   Stir in the arugula and toss it over medium heat until it wilts; about 30 seconds.

5.   Remove the dish from the heat and stir in the remaining half teaspoon of oil and lemon zest.

Note: You can reheat this recipe the next day, and it will still taste great. Alternatively, you can serve it as a cold salad. Allow it come to room temperature and then toss it, adding just a bit of red wine or balsamic vinegar.

Creamy Mushroom And Chicken Stew Crockpot

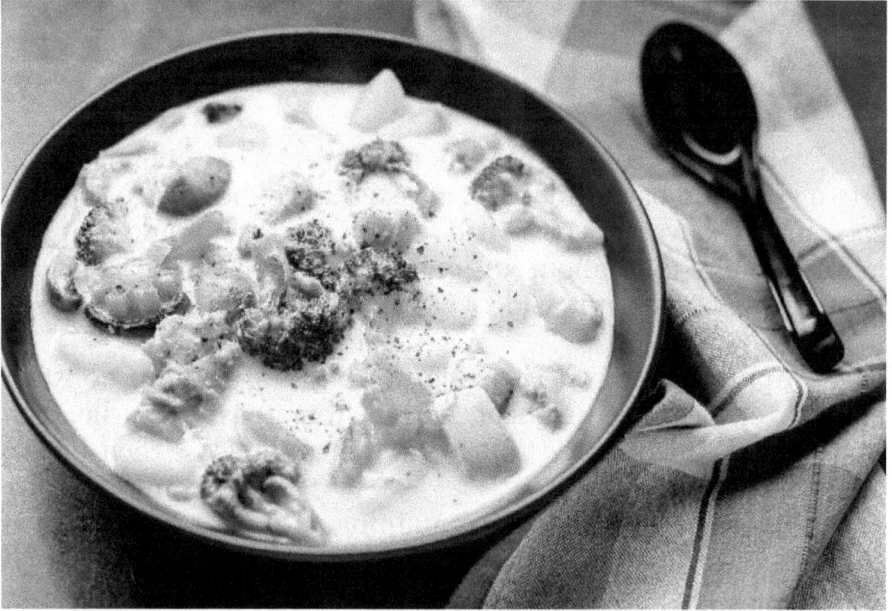

SmartPoints value: Green plan - 2SP, Blue plan - 2SP, Purple plan - 2SP

Total Time: 4hr 20min, Prep time: 10 min, Cooking time: 4hr 10mins,

Serves: 4

Nutritional value: Calories – 278, Carbs – 24.2g, Fat – 4.2g, Protein – 32g

The mushroom and chicken stew crockpot is a fantastic low-calorie dinner idea. It's a healthy and easy slow cooker recipe with great taste.

Ingredients

- Chicken breast (skinless) - 1 lb

- Baby portabella mushroom (sliced) - 8 oz

- Onion (finely chopped) - 1 piece

- Carrots (cut into matchsticks) - 1/2 cup

- Peas (fresh or frozen) - 1/2 cup

- Celery (chopped) - 2 stalks

- Mushroom seasoning (powdered) - 2 tbsp

- Chicken broth (fat-free) - 2 cups

- Sour cream (fat-free, at room temp) - 1 cup

- Garlic (minced) - 3 cloves

- Salt (1 tsp)

- Pepper (1/2 tsp)

Instructions

1.   Combine all ingredients in a crockpot except the sour cream.

2.   For 4- 6 hrs., cook on low heat.
3.   For about 5 minutes, stir in sour cream, and warm until it is thoroughly heated. Serve immediately.

Smashed Avocado And Egg Toast

SmartPoints value: Green plan – 6SP, Blue plan – 4SP, Purple plan - 4SP

Total Time: 7 min, Prep time: 5 min, Cooking time: 2 min, Serves: 1

Nutritional value: Calories – 214.0, Carbs - 16.4g, Fat – 14.2g, Protein - 8.4g

Ingredients

- Avocado - ¼ item(s), medium-sized, ripe but still a touch firm

- Light whole-grain bread - 1 slice(s)

- Whole hard-boiled egg(s) - 1 item(s), sliced

- Table salt - 1 pinch

- Crushed red pepper flakes - 1 pinch

- Black pepper - 1 pinch

Instructions

1. Place one slice of bread on a clean plate.

2.   Top with a portion of peeled avocado and gently smash with a knife or fork.

3.   Cut hard-boiled egg in half and place each half on the bread.

4.   Gently smash egg and mix with smashed avocado. Season the bread to taste with salt, pepper, and red pepper flakes.

5.   Cover with another slice of bread and place in a flat-sitting electric bread toaster.

6.   Remove smashed avocado and egg toast from the toaster once the "ready" light comes on.

Sweet Pineapple and Strawberry Salsa with Yogurt

The best salsas sometimes don't contain tomatoes, and this sweet pineapple and strawberry salsa with yogurt recipe is a good example.

I've added coconut flakes to this recipe to give a pleasant taste of fresh fruit. SmartPoints value: Green plan – 3SP, Blue plan – 2SP, Purple plan - 2SP Total Time: 8 min, Prep time: 4 min, Cooking time: 4 min Serves: 1 Nutritional value: Calories - 30.9, Carbs - 7.4g, Fat - 0.4g, Protein - 0.4g
Ingredients

- Strawberries - 3 medium-sized, diced - fresh mint leaves - 1 tsp (chopped)
- Pineapple - ½ cup(s),
- Golden species (diced)
- Plain fat-free Greek yogurt - ½ cup(s)
- Lime zest - ⅛ tsp (grated)
- Unsweetened coconut flakes - 1 Tbsp (toasted)
- Coconut flakes – 3 Tbsp

Instructions

Dice strawberries, pineapple, mint, and lime zest into a small bowl, all mixed.

Add yogurt and speckle with coconut. You can also spoon the yogurt into a glass dish and top it with fruit and coconut.

Creamy Banana French Toast Casserole

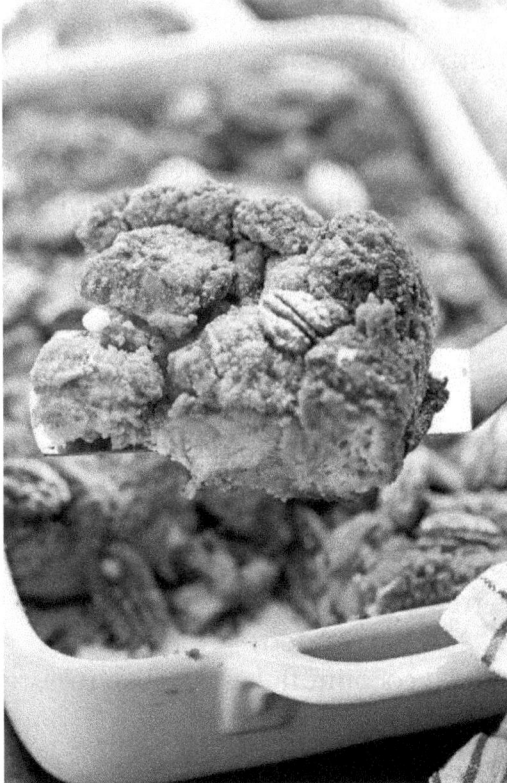

You can give a bright flavor to this creamy casserole and also keep the banana from turning black by adding a small quantity of lemon juice.

SmartPoints value: Green plan – 7SP, Blue plan – 6SP, Purple plan - 6SP

Total Time: 55 min, Prep time: 20 min, Cooking time: 35 min, Serves: 12

Nutritional value:

Calories - 489, Carbs - 68.7g, Fat - 18g, Protein - 15.4g

Ingredients

- Cooking spray - 5 spray(s)
- Whole wheat/oatmeal bread - 12 slice(s), cut into quarters (about 1 oz per slice)
- Neufchâtel cheese - 4 oz, (1/3-less-fat cream cheese)
- 2% reduced-fat milk - 1 cup(s)
- Maple syrup - ½ cup(s)
- Egg(s) - 6 large
- Banana(s) - 4 medium-sized, ripe (divided)
- Fresh lemon juice - 2 tsp
- Rum - 1 Tbsp
- Ground cinnamon - ½ tsp
- Vanilla extract - 1 tsp
- Ground nutmeg - ½ tsp
- Table salt - ¼ tsp
- Powdered sugar - 3 Tbsp

Instructions

1. Get a clean 13 inches by 9 inches baking dish and coat it with cooking spray.

2. Stand quarter portions of bread up in the prepared dish, so it lines the sides and bottom in a single layer — Preheat the oven to 350°F.

3. Place the cheese, milk, and syrup in a blender.
4. Add eggs, two bananas, rum, vanilla, juice, nutmeg, cinnamon, and salt to the blender.
5. Allow the blending process to Dash until the mixture is smooth.

6. Gently pour the mixture over the bread and press those on the sides of the baking dish into the egg mixture, making sure it is completely submerged.

7.	Refrigerate the dish for 30 minutes after covering with foil.
8.	Preheat the oven again to 350°F. Just before baking, thinly slice the remaining two bananas and put the slices in between pieces of bread.
9.	Cover the dish with new foil and bake for 25 minutes. Remove the

foil and continue baking until the color is golden brown. Set for about 10 minutes more, then sprinkle the top with powdered sugar. Slice the casserole into 12 pieces and serve immediately.

Note: You can serve with fresh berries if you desire.

Fried Egg With Asparagus-Potato Hash

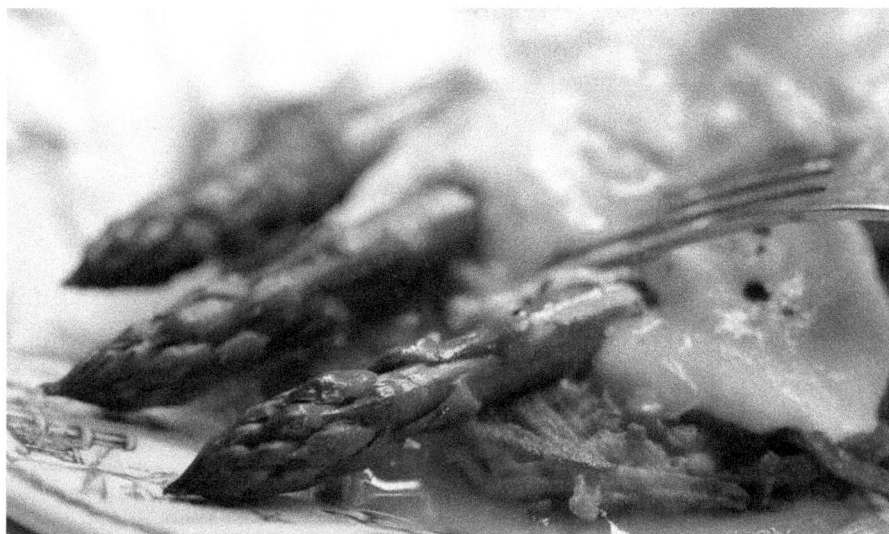

Eggs look great with asparagus in this fantastic breakfast recipe. To effortlessly prepare asparagus so that the cooking will be fast and be tender, bend the spears near the tail until the woody part breaks off. You can also use the points of the spears and reserve the middle of the asparagus stalks for another preparation like a veggie stir-fry or steamed in a green salad. You should microwave the potato and then sauté it. Microwaving ensures that the interior is soft, with a crisped, browned exterior, a perfectly hashed topping to your egg.

SmartPoints value: Green plan – 7SP, Blue plan – 5SP, Purple plan - 1SP Total Time: 22 min, Prep time: 12 min, Cooking time: 10 min, Serves: 1 Nutritional value: Calories - 319, Carbs - 38.4g, Fat - 8g, Protein - 11.5g Ingredients

- Uncooked red potato(es) - 1 medium-sized, pierced severally with a fork
- Uncooked asparagus - 4 spear(s), medium-sized, trimmed, diagonally sliced 1/2-inch thick (1/2 cup)

- Uncooked scallion(s) - 1 small (sliced)
- Olive oil - 1 tsp
- Table salt - ¼ tsp
- Fresh thyme - 1 tsp (chopped)
- Egg(s) - 1 large, cooked sunny-side up
- Black pepper - 1 pinch

Instructions

1. Microwave potato for about 3-4 minutes and cut into small dice.

2.   Heat the oil in a medium-sized, nonstick skillet over a medium to high heat.

3.   Add the asparagus and diced potato to the oil
4.   Cook, occasionally stirring, until the diced potatoes are browned, and asparagus is crisp-tender, about 4 minutes.
5.   Add the scallion and thyme; keep stirring until scallion wilts, about 30 seconds.
6.   Season with salt and pepper, then serve with egg.

Greek-Style Scrambled Eggs

If you need a quick and easy weeknight dish, you can prepare these scrambled eggs within 20 minutes. These eggs make a perfect one-dish meal, loaded with various flavors that include butter beans, chicken chorizo sausage, grape tomatoes, and onions.

To make this meal vegetarian, add soy-based breakfast sausage. You can use lentils in place of butter beans if you can't find them.

Prevent overcooking by turning off the heat before the eggs are all the way cooked.

SmartPoints value: Green plan – 8SP, Blue plan – 3SP, Purple plan - 3SP Total Time: 20 min, Prep time: 12 min, Cooking time: 8 min, Serves: 1 Nutritional value: Calories - 221, Carbs - 5.1g, Fat - 10.3g, Protein - 21.0g Ingredients

- Cooked chicken chorizo sausage - 1½ oz (diced)
- Cooking spray - 5 spray(s)
- Canned butter beans - ¼ cup(s), rinsed and drained
- Crumbled feta cheese - 1 Tbsp
- Uncooked onion(s) - ¼ cup(s) (chopped)
- Grape tomatoes - 6 medium-sized (halved)
- Egg(s) - 2 large
- Black pepper - 1 pinch, or add to taste
- Table salt - 1 pinch, or add to taste
- Dill - 1 Tbsp, chopped

Instructions

1.   Coat a medium-sized nonstick skillet with nonstick spray.

2.   Add chicken chorizo and onion, then cook over medium heat, occasionally stirring, until lightly browned, about 5 minutes.

3.   Add tomatoes and beans, then stir until the tomatoes start to soften, about 1 minute.

4.   Push the mixture to one side of the skillet and add eggs to the other side.

5.   Scramble the eggs until softly set, 1-2 minutes.

6.   Turn in the chorizo mixture and season with salt and pepper, then sprinkle with dill and feta.

Italian Turkey Sausage And Vegetable Omelet

You can prepare this hearty 20-minute entrée for breakfast, lunch, or dinner, and it is perfect for one-person cooking.

The omelet fills with chicken sausage, onion, mushrooms, and roasted red peppers, then finished with salty Pecorino Romano cheese, which is chopped parsley. This addition injects freshness and color. Italian sausages come in several varieties that are sweet and spicy, so use your favorite in this recipe. When preparing omelets, it's good to practice to cook all the fillings and get them ready to go before you start cooking the eggs, since the cooking process is a quick one that takes only a couple minutes per omelet.

SmartPoints value: Green plan - 6SP, Blue plan - 2SP, Purple plan - 2SP Total Time: 20 min, Prep time: 10 min, Cooking time: 10 min, Serves: 1 Nutritional value: Calories - 292.3, Carbs - 5.1g, Fat - 21.4g, Protein - 22.9g Ingredients

- Cooked chicken or turkey sausage(s) - 1½ oz, Italian-variety, chopped
- Fresh edible mushroom(s) - ¾ cup(s), chopped
- Fresh parsley - ½ Tbsp, chopped
- Uncooked onion(s) - ¼ cup(s), chopped
- Cooking spray - 4 spray(s)
- Egg(s) - 2 large, beaten with a pinch of salt and pepper
- Grated Pecorino Romano cheese - 1½ Tbsp
- Chopped and roasted red peppers (packed in water) - ¼ cup(s)

Instructions

1.   Coat a small-sized omelet pan with cooking spray and heat over medium flame.

2.   Add the sausage, mushroom, and onion, then cook, frequently stirring, until the onions soften, 5 minutes. Remove the cooked omelet from pan to a bowl and stir in roasted pepper, then set aside.

3.   Wipe the pan clean with a paper towel.
4.   Put off heat, coat the pan again with cooking spray, and heat over medium flame.
5.   Add the beaten eggs and swirl to spread egg over the pan.
6.   Cook it until the bottom is done and the top is nearly cooked for about 3 minutes.
7.   Top the omelet with chicken sausage mixture and sprinkle with cheese.
8.   Fold the omelet over and cook for 1-2 minutes more. Serve it sprinkled with parsley.

Chinese-Style Zucchini With Ginger

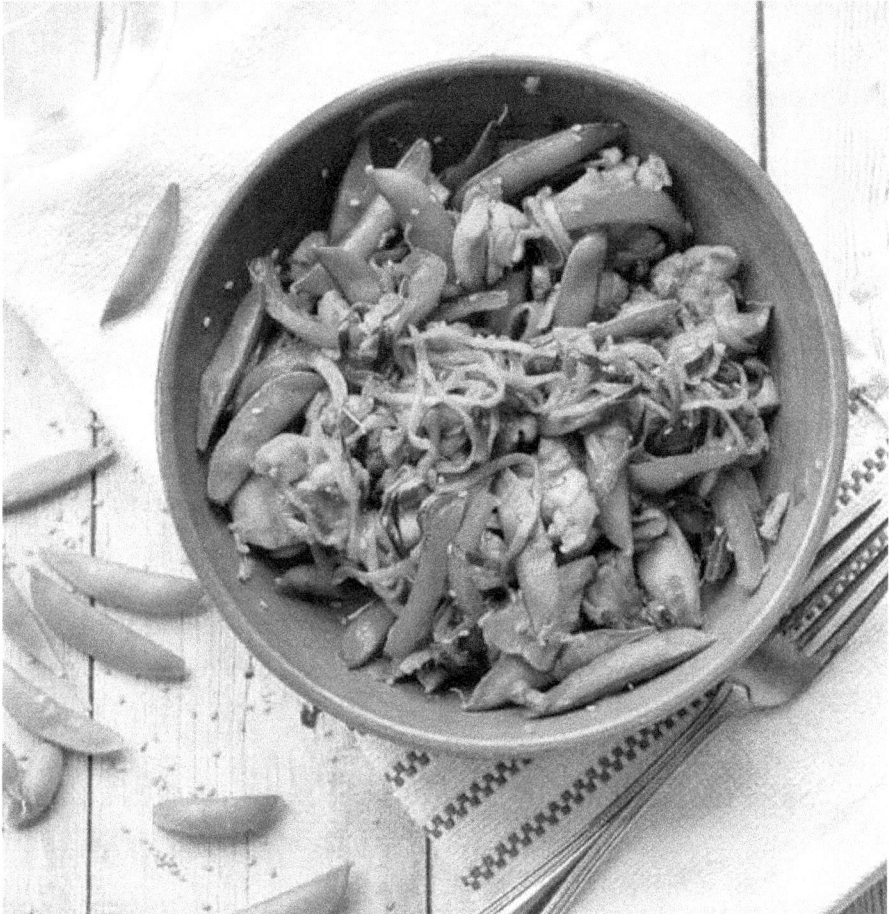

Servings per container - 10

Prep Total - 10 min

Serving Size 2/3 cup (55g)

Nutritional Facts

Total Fat 8g

Total Carbohydrate 37g

Protein 3g

Sodium 160mg

Ingredients:

- 1 teaspoon oil
- 1 lb. zucchini cut into 1/4-inch slices
- 1/2 cup vegetarian broth
- 2 teaspoon light soy sauce
- 1 teaspoon dry sherry
- 1 teaspoon toasted sesame oil

Instructions:

1.   Heat a large wok or heavy skillets over high heat until very hot then add the oil. When the oil is hot, add the zucchini and ginger.

2.   Stir-fry 1 minute.
3.   Add the broth, soy sauce, and sherry.
4.   Stir-fry over high heat until the broth cooks down a bit and the zucchini is crisp-tender.
5.   Remove from the heat, sprinkle with sesame oil and serve.

Breakfast Super Antioxidant Berry Smoothie

servings per container - 5

Prep Total - 10 min

Serving Size - 4 cup (20g)

Nutritional Facts

Total Fat 2g

Sodium 7mg

Total Carbohydrate 20g

Protein 3g

Ingredients

- 1 cup of filtered water
- 1 whole orange, peeled, de-seeded & cut into chunks
- 2 cups frozen raspberries or blackberries
- 1 Tablespoon goji berries
- 1 1/2 Tablespoons hemp seeds or plant-based protein powder
- 2 cups leafy greens (parsley, spinach, or kale)

Instructions:

Blend on high until smooth

Serve and drink immediately

Cucumber Tomato Surprise

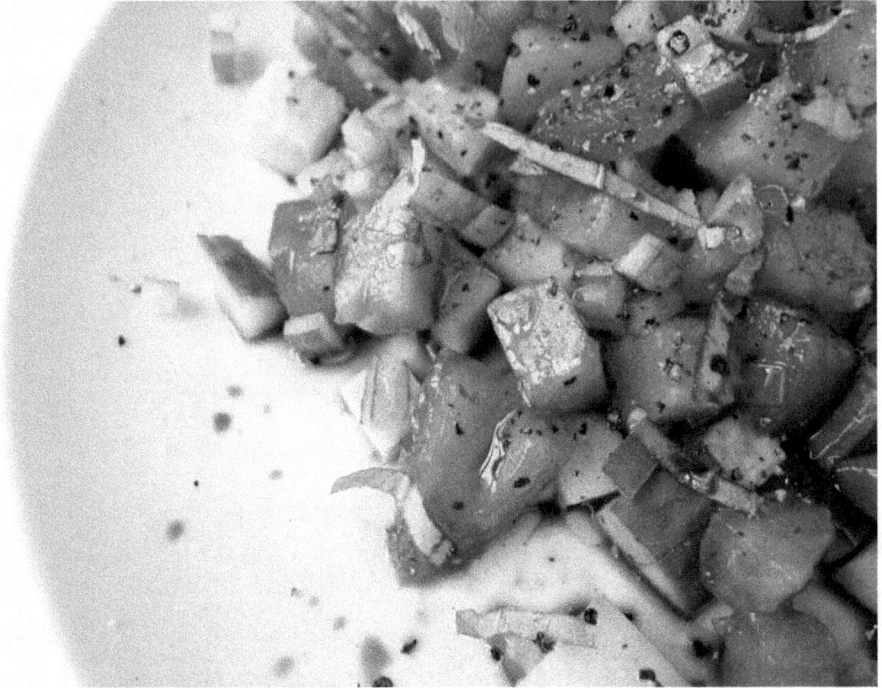

servings per container - 5

Prep Total - 10 min
Serving Size 2/3 cup (55g)

Nutritional Facts

Total Fat 20g

Total Carbohydrate 14g

Total Sugar 2g

Protein 7g

Ingredients

- Chopped 1 medium of tomato
- 1 small cucumber peeled in stripes and chopped
- 1 large avocado cut into cubes
- 1 half of a lemon or lime squeezed
- ½1 tsp. Himalayan or Real salt
- 1 Teaspoon of original olive oil, MCT or coconut oil

Instructions:

1.   Mix everything together and enjoy

2.   This dish tastes even better after sitting for 40 – 60 minutes

3.   Blend into a soup if desired.

Avocado Nori Rolls

Nutritional Facts

servings per container   10
Prep Total   10 min
Serving Size 2/3 cup (70g)
Amount per serving 15
Calories
          % Daily Value
Total Fat 2g   10%
Saturated Fat 1g   9%
Trans Fat 10g   -
Cholesterol   1%
Sodium 70mg   5%
Total Carbohydrate 22g   40%
Dietary Fiber 4g   2%
Total Sugar 12g   -
Protein 3g
Vitamin C 2mcg   2%
Calcium 260mg   7%
Iron 8mg   2%
Potassium 235mg   4%

Ingredients

- 2 sheets of raw or toasted sushi nori

- 1 large Romaine leaf cut in half down the length of the spine

- 2 Teaspoon of spicy miso paste

- 1 avocado, peeled and sliced

- ½ red, yellow or orange bell pepper, julienned
- ½ cucumber, peeled, seeded and julienned
- ½ cup raw sauerkraut
- ½ carrot, beet or zucchini, shredded
- 1 cup alfalfa or favorite green sprouts
- 1 small bowl of water for sealing roll

Instructions:

1.   Place a sheet of nori on a sushi rolling mat or washcloth, lining it up at the end closest to you.

2.   Place the Romaine leaf on the edge of the nori with the spine closest to you.
3.   Spread Spicy Miso Paste on the Romaine
4.   Line the leaf with all ingredients in descending order, placing

sprouts on last

5.   Roll the Nori sheet away from you, tucking the ingredients in with your fingers, and seal the roll with water or Spicy Miso Paste. Slice the roll into 6 or 8 rounds.

Maple Ginger Pancakes

Nutritional Facts

servings per container   4
Prep Total   10 min
Serving Size 2/3 cup (20g)
Amount per serving 20
Calories

            % Daily Value
Total Facts 10g   10%
Saturated Fat 0g   7%
Trans Fat 2g -
Cholesterol   3%
Sodium 10mg   2%
Total Carbohydrate 7g   3%
Dietary Fiber 2g   4%
Total Sugar 1g   -
Protein 3g
Vitamin C 2mcg   10%
Calcium 260mg   20%
Iron 8mg   30%
Potassium 235mg   6%

Ingredients

- 1 or 2 cup flour
- 1 tablespoonful baking powder
- 1/2 tablespoonful kosher salt
- 1/4 tablespoonful ground ginger
- 1/4 table spoonful pumpkin pie spice
- 1/3 cup maple syrup
- 2/4 cup water

- minced 1/4 cup + 1 tablespoonful crystallized ginger slices together

Instructions:

1.   In a neat bowl mix together the first five recipes

2.   Add flour with syrup with water and stir together, after that add in the chopped ginger & stir until-just-combined.
3.   Heat your frying pan and coat with a nonstick cooking spray
4.   Pour in 1/4 cup of the batter and allow to heat until it form bubbles. Allow to cook until browned
5.   Serve warm & topped with a slathering of vegan butter, a splash of maple syrup, and garnished with chopped candied ginger.

Chewy Chocolate Chip Cookies

Nutritional Facts

servings per container   10
Prep Total   10 min
Serving Size 2/3 cup (40g)
Amount per serving 10
Calories

         % Daily Value
Total Fat 10g 2%
Saturated Fat 1g   5%
Trans Fat 0g -
Cholesterol   15%
Sodium 120mg   8%
Total Carbohydrate 21g   10%
Dietary Fiber 4g   1%
Total Sugar 1g   0%
Protein 6g
Vitamin C 2mcg   7%
Calcium 210mg   51%
Iron 8mg   1%
Potassium 235mg   10%

Ingredients

- 1 cup vegan butter, softened
  - ½ cup white sugar
- ½ cup brown sugar
- ¼ cup dairy-free milk
- 1 teaspoon vanilla
- 2 ¼ cups flour
- ½ teaspoon salt
- 1 teaspoon baking soda
- 12 ounces dairy-free chocolate chips

Instructions:

1.   Preheat oven to 350°F.

2.   In a large bowl, mix the butter, white sugar, and brown sugar until light and fluffy. Slowly stir in the dairy-free milk and then add the vanilla to make a creamy mixture.

3.   In a separate bowl, combine the flour, salt, and baking soda.

4.   You need to add this dry mixture to the liquid mixture and stir well. Fold in the chocolate chips.

5.   Drop small spoonful of the batter onto non-stick cookie sheets and bake for 9 minutes.

Fudge Brownies

Nutritional Facts

servings per container   9
Prep Total   10 min
Serving Size 2/3 cup (70g)
Amount per serving 10
Calories

	% Daily Value	
Total Fat 20g	2%	
Saturated Fat 2g	10%	
Trans Fat 4g -		
Cholesterol 10%		
Sodium 50mg	12%	
Total Carbohydrate 7g		20%
Dietary Fiber 4g	7%	
Total Sugar 12g	-	
Protein 3g		
Vitamin C 2mcg	19%	

Calcium 260mg   20%
Iron 8mg   8%
Potassium 235mg   6%

Ingredients

Instructions:

1.   Preheat oven to 350°F and grease a 9 x 13-inch baking pan.

2.   Add dry ingredients in a mixing bowl. Whisk together wet ingredients and fold into the dry ingredients.
3.   If desired, add half the chocolate chips and chopped walnuts to the mix. Pour mixture into the prepared pan and sprinkle with remaining chocolate chips and walnuts, if using.
4.   For fudge-like brownies, bake for 20-25 minutes. For cake-like brownies, bake 25-30 minutes. Let the brownies cool slightly before serving.

Pomegranate Quinoa Porridge

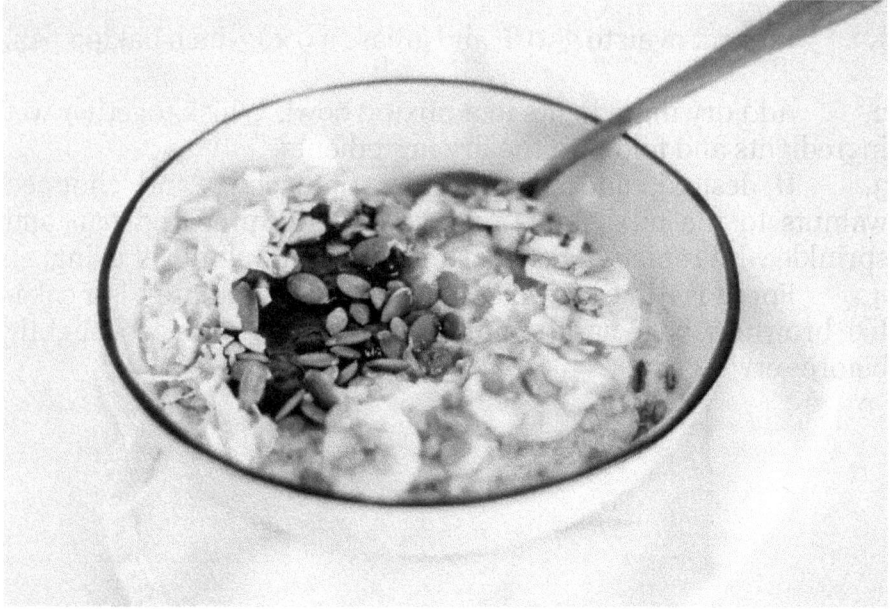

Nutritional Facts

servings per container   4

Prep Total   10 min

Serving Size 2/3 cup (40g)

Amount per serving 22
Calories

        % Daily Value

Total Fat 12g 20%

Saturated Fat 2g   4%

Trans Fat 01g   1.22%

Cholesterol   22%

Sodium 170mg   10%

Total Carbohydrate 34g   22%

Dietary Fiber 5g   14%

Total Sugar 7g   -

Protein 3g

Vitamin C 2mcg   10%

Calcium 260mg   20%

Iron 0mg   40%

Potassium 235mg   6%

Ingredients

- 1 1/2 cup quinoa flakes
- 2 1/2 teaspoons cinnamon
- 1 teaspoon vanilla extract
- 10 organic pDashes, pitted and cut into 1/4's
- 1 pomegranate pulp
- 1/4 cup desiccated coconut
- Stewed apples

- Coconut flakes to garnish

Instructions:

1.   Gently place quinoa & almond milk into saucepan, & stir on medium to low heat for 9 minutes, until it smooth

2.   Include cinnamon, desiccated coconut & vanilla extract & taste

3.   Pit pDashes & cut into quarters include to porridge stir in well

4.   Serve into individual bowls

5.   Add a scoop of stewed apple (kindly view recipe below), pomegranates, pDashes & coconut flakes

6. Ready to eat!

Stewed apples

1.   Peel, core, slice apples and place into a saucepan with water

2.   Cook apples on medium heat, until extremely soft
3.   Remove from heat, drain & mash apples
4.   Ready to serve and enjoy your breakfast!

Cinnamon and Coconut Porridge

Serving: 4

Prep Time: 5 minutes

Cook Time: 5 minutes

Ingredients:

- 1 cup water
- 1/2 cup 36-percent low-fat cream
- ½ cup unsweetened dried coconut, shredded 1 tablespoon oat bran
- 1 tablespoon flaxseed meal
- 1/2 tablespoon almond butter
- 1 ½ teaspoons stevia
- ½ teaspoon cinnamon
- Toppings, such as blueberries or banana slices

How To:

1.   Add the ingredients to alittle pot and blend well until fully incorporated

2.   Transfer the pot to your stove over medium-low heat and convey the combination to a slow boil.
3.   Stir well and take away from the warmth .
4.   Divide the mixture into equal servings and allow them to sit for 10 minutes.
5.   Top together with your desired toppings and enjoy!

Nutrition (Per Serving)

Calories: 171

Fat: 16g

Protein: 2g

Carbohydrates: 8g

Coconut Porridge

Serving: 2

Prep Time: 15 minutes

Cook Time: Nil

Ingredients:

- 2 tablespoons coconut flour
- 2 tablespoons vanilla protein powder
- 3 tablespoons Golden Flaxseed meal
- 1 ½ cups almond milk, unsweetened
- Powdered Erythritol

How To:

1.   Take a bowl and blend within the flaxseed meal, protein powder, coconut flour and blend well.

2.   Add the combination to the saucepan (placed over medium heat).

3.   Add almond milk and stir, let the mixture thicken.
4.   Add your required amount of sweetener and serve.
5.   Enjoy!

Nutrition (Per Serving)

Calories: 259

Fat: 13g

Carbohydrates: 5g

Protein: 16g

Cinnamon Pear Oatmeal

Serving: 2

Prep Time: 10 minutes

Cook Time: 15 minutes

Ingredients:

- 3 cups water
- 1 cup steel-cut oats
- 1 tablespoon cinnamon powder
- 1 cup pear, cored and peeled, cubed

How To:

1.   Take a pot and add the water, oats, cinnamon, pear and toss well.

2.   Bring it to simmer over medium heat.
3.   Let it cook for quarter-hour , and divide into two bowls.
4.   Enjoy!

Nutrition (Per Serving)

Calories: 171

Fat: 5g

Carbohydrates: 11g

Protein: 6g

Banana and Walnut Bowl

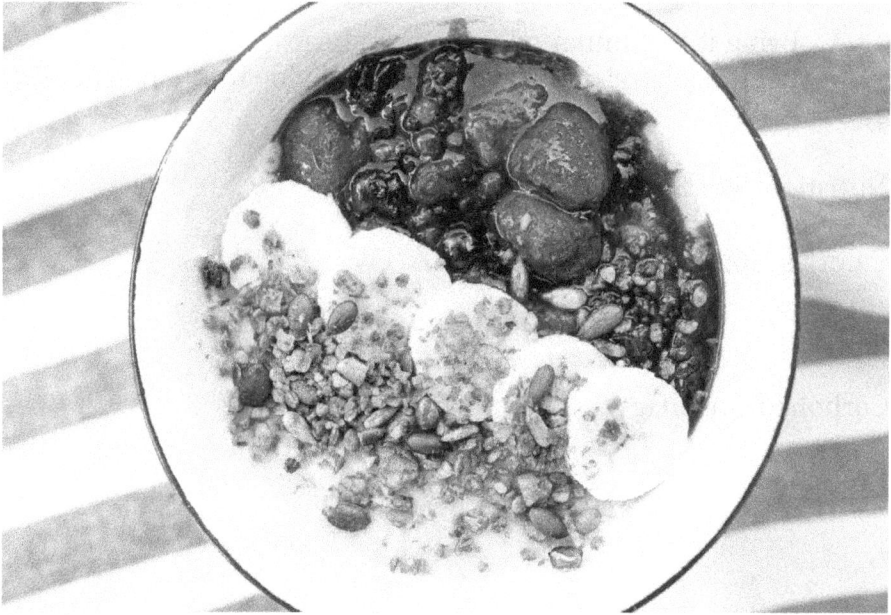

Serving: 4

Prep Time: 10 minutes

Cook Time: 15 minutes

Ingredients:

- 2 cups water
- 1 cup steel-cut oats
- 1 cup almond milk
- ¼ cup walnuts, chopped
- 2 tablespoons chia seeds
- 2 bananas, peeled and mashed
- 1 teaspoon vanilla flavoring

How To:

1.   Take a pot and add all ingredients, toss well.

2.   Bring it to simmer over medium heat.
3.   Let it cook for quarter-hour , and divide into 4 bowls.
4.   Enjoy!

Nutrition (Per Serving)

Calories: 162

Fat: 4g

Carbohydrates: 11g

Protein: 4g

Scrambled Pesto Eggs

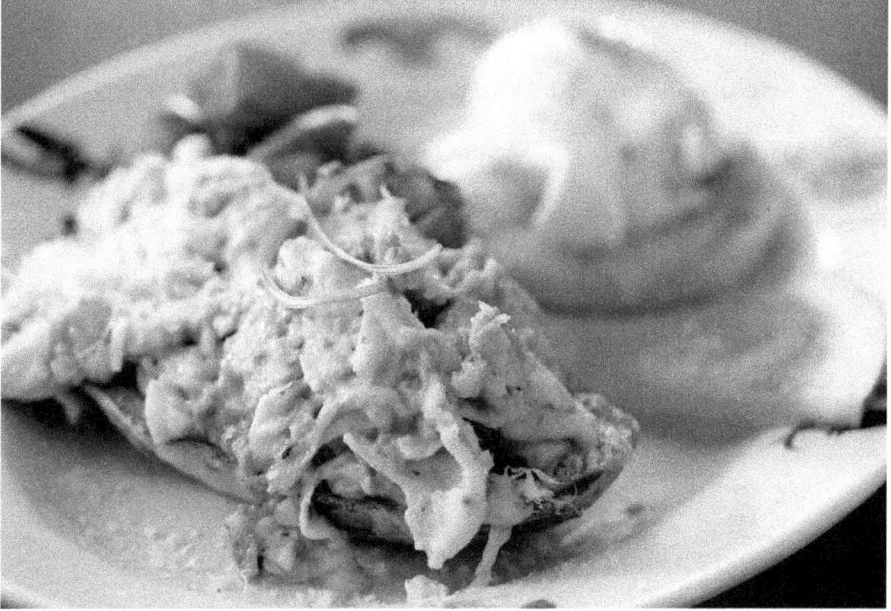

Serving: 2

Prep Time: 5 minutes

Cook Time: 5 minutes

Ingredients:

- 2 large whole eggs
- 1/2 tablespoon almond butter
- 1/2 tablespoon pesto
- 1 tablespoon creamed coconut
- almond milk

- Sunflower seeds and pepper as needed

How To:

1.   Take a bowl and crack open your eggs.

2.   Season with a pinch of sunflower seeds and pepper.
3.   Pour eggs into a pan.
4.   Add almond butter and introduce heat.
5.   Cook on low heat and gently add pesto.
6.   Once the eggs are cooked and scrambled, remove from the warmth.

7.   Spoon in coconut milk and blend well.
8.   activate the warmth and cook on LOW for a short time until you've

got a creamy texture.

9. Serve and enjoy!

Nutrition (Per Serving)

Calories: 467

Fat: 41g

Carbohydrates: 3g

Protein: 20g

Barley Porridge

Serving: 4

Prep Time: 5 minutes

Cook Time: 25 minutes

Ingredients:

- 1 cup barley
- 1 cup wheat berries
- 2 cups unsweetened almond milk
- 2 cups water
- Toppings, such as hazelnuts, honey, berry, etc.

How To:

1.   Take a medium saucepan and place it over medium-high heat.

2.   Place barley, almond milk, wheat berries, water and convey to a boil.
3.   Lower the warmth to low and simmer for 25 minutes.
4.   Divide amongst serving bowls and top together with your desired toppings.
5.   Serve and enjoy!

Nutrition (Per Serving)

Calories: 295

Fat: 8g

Carbohydrates: 56g

Protein: 6g

Olive Cherry Bites

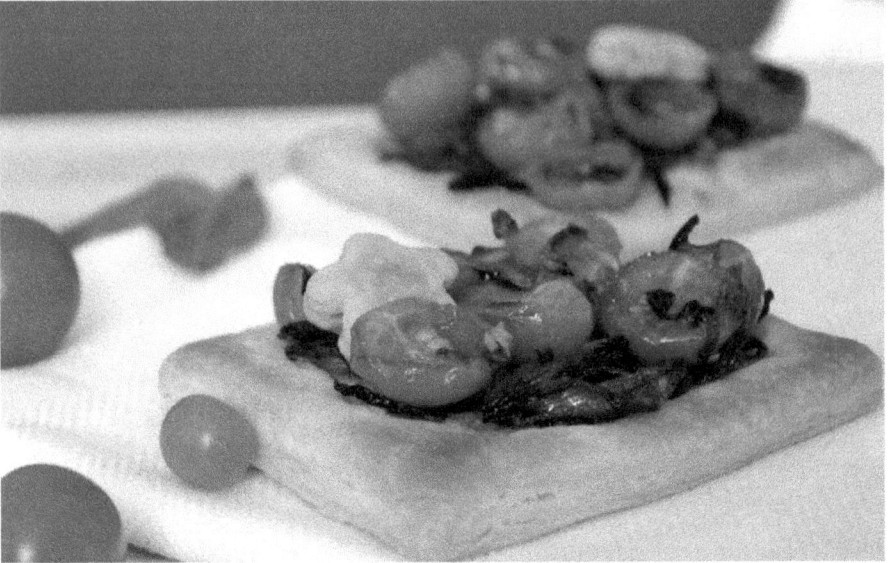

Serving: 30

Prep Time: 15 minutes

Cook Time: Nil

Ingredients:

- 24 cherry tomatoes, halved

- 24 black olives, pitted

- 24 feta cheese cubes

- 24 toothpick/decorative skewers

How To:

1.   Use a toothpick or skewer and thread feta cheese, black olives, cherry tomato halves therein order.

2.   Repeat until all the ingredients are used.
3.   Arrange during a serving platter.
4.   Serve and enjoy!

Nutrition (Per Serving)

Calories: 57

Fat: 5g

Carbohydrates: 2g

Protein: 2g

Roasted Herb Crackers

Serving: 75 Crackers

Prep Time: 10 minutes

Cook Time: 120 minutes

Ingredients:

- ¼ cup avocado oil
- 10 celery sticks
- 1 sprig fresh rosemary, stem discarded
- 2 sprigs fresh thyme, stems discarded
- 2 tablespoons apple cider vinegar
- 1 teaspoon Himalayan sunflower seeds
- 3 cups ground flaxseeds

How To:

1.   Preheat your oven to 225 degrees F.

2.   Line a baking sheet with parchment paper and keep it on the side.

3.   Add oil, herbs, celery, vinegar, sunflower seeds to a kitchen appliance and pulse until you've got a good mixture.
4.   Add flax and puree.
5.   Let it sit for 2-3 minutes.
6.   Transfer batter to your prepared baking sheet and spread evenly, dig cracker shapes.
7.   Bake for hour , flip and bake for hour more.
8.   Enjoy!

Nutrition (Per Serving)

Calories: 34

Fat: 5g

Carbohydrates: 1g

Protein: 1.3g

Banana Steel Oats

Serving: 3

Prep Time: 10 minutes

Cook Time: 15 minutes

Ingredients:

- 1 small banana
- 1 cup almond milk
- ¼ teaspoon cinnamon, ground
- ½ cup rolled oats
- 1 tablespoon honey

How To:

1.   Take a saucepan and add half the banana, whisk in almond milk, ground cinnamon.

2.   Season with sunflower seeds.
3.   Stir until the banana is mashed well, bring the mixture to a boil and stir in oats.
4.   Reduce heat to medium-low and simmer for 5-7 minutes until the oats are tender.
5.   Dice the remaining half banana and placed on the highest of the oatmeal.
6.   Enjoy!

Nutrition (Per Serving)

Calories: 358

Fat: 6g

Carbohydrates: 76g

Protein: 7g

Swiss Chard Omelet

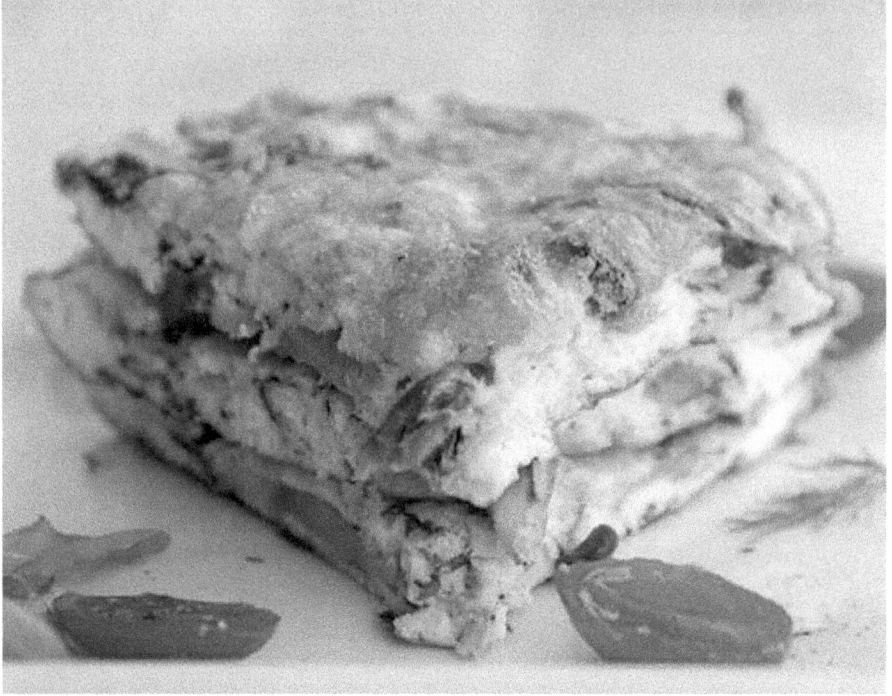

Serving: 2

Prep Time: 5 minutes

Cook Time: 5 minutes

Ingredients:

- 2 eggs, lightly beaten
- 2 cups Swiss chard, sliced
- 1 tablespoon almond butter
- ½ teaspoon sunflower seeds
- Fresh pepper

How To:

1.   Take a non-stick frypan and place it over medium-low heat.

2.   Once the almond butter melts, add Swiss chard and stir-cook for two minutes.

3.   Pour the eggs into the pan and gently stir them into Swiss chard.

4.   Season with garlic sunflower seeds and pepper.
5.   Cook for two minutes.
6.   Serve and enjoy!

Nutrition (Per Serving)

Calories: 260

Fat: 21g

Carbohydrates: 4g

Protein: 14g

Hearty Pineapple Oatmeal

Serving: 5

Prep Time: 10 minutes

Cook Time: 4-8 hours

Ingredients:

- 1 cup steel-cut oats

- 4 cups unsweetened almond milk

- 2 medium apples, sliced

- 1 teaspoon coconut oil

- 1 teaspoon cinnamon

- ¼ teaspoon nutmeg

- 2 tablespoons maple syrup, unsweetened
- A drizzle of lemon juice

How To:

1.   Add listed ingredients to a pan and blend well.

2.   Cook on very low flame for 8 hours/or on high flame for 4 hours.

3.   Gently stir.
4.   Add your required toppings.
5.   Serve and enjoy!
6.   Store within the fridge for later use; confirm to feature a splash of almond milk after re-heating for added flavor.

Nutrition (Per Serving)

Calories: 180

Fat: 5g

Carbohydrates: 31g

Protein: 5g

Zingy Onion and Thyme Crackers

Serving: 75 crackers

Prep Time: 15 minutes

Cooking Time: 120 minutes

Ingredients:

- 1 garlic clove, minced

- 1 cup sweet onion, coarsely chopped

- 2 teaspoons fresh thyme leaves

- ¼ cup avocado oil

- ¼ teaspoon garlic powder

- Freshly ground black pepper

- ¼ cup sunflower seeds

- 1 ½ cups roughly ground flax seeds

How To:

1. Preheat your oven to 225 degrees F.

2. Line two baking sheets with parchment paper and keep it on the side.

3. Add garlic, onion, thyme, oil, sunflower seeds, and pepper to a kitchen appliance .

4. Add sunflower and flax seeds, pulse until pureed.

5. Transfer the batter to prepared baking sheets and spread evenly, dig crackers

6. Bake for hour .

7. Remove parchment paper and flip crackers, bake for an additional hour.

8. If crackers are thick, it'll take longer .

9. Remove from oven and allow them to cool.

10. Enjoy!

Nutrition (Per Serving)

Total Carbs: 0.8g

Fiber: 0.2g

Protein: 0.4g

Fat: 2.7g

Crunchy Flax and Almond Crackers

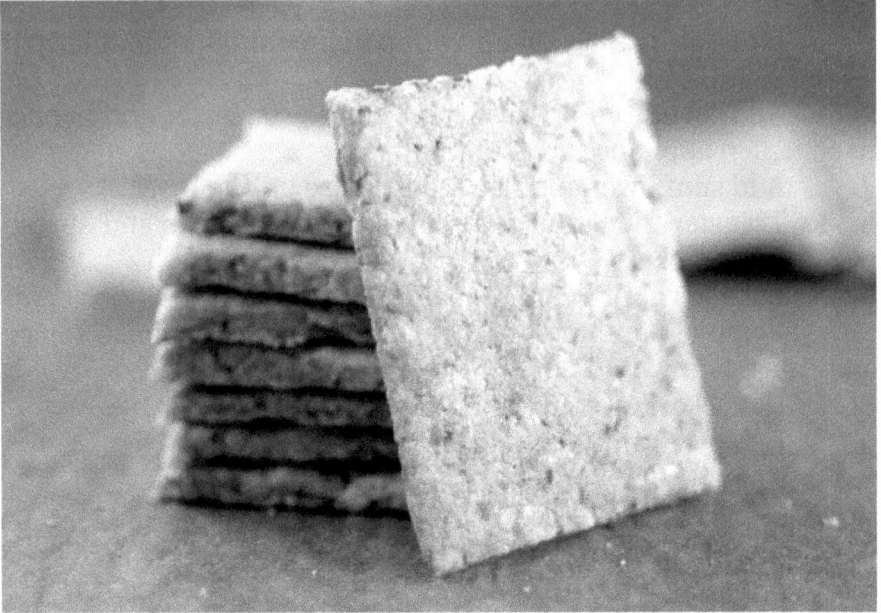

Serving: 20-24 crackers

Prep Time: 15 minutes

Cooking Time: 60 minutes

Ingredients:

- ½ cup ground flaxseeds
- ½ cup almond flour
- 1 tablespoon coconut flour
- 2 tablespoons shelled hemp seeds
- ¼ teaspoon sunflower seeds
- 1 egg white
- 2 tablespoons unsalted almond butter, melted

How To:

1.   Preheat your oven to 300 degrees F.

2.   Line a baking sheet with parchment paper, keep it on the side.

3.   Add flax, almond, coconut flour, hemp seed, seeds to a bowl and blend .
4.   Add albumen and melted almond butter, mix until combined.
5.   Transfer dough to a sheet of parchment paper and canopy with another sheet of paper.
6.   Roll out dough.
7.   dig crackers and bake for hour .
8.   allow them to cool and enjoy!

Nutrition (Per Serving)

Total Carbs: 1.2

Fiber: 1g

Protein: 2g

Fat: 6g

Basil and Tomato Baked Eggs

Serving: 2

Prep Time: 10 minutes

Cook Time: 15 minutes

Ingredients:

- 1/2 garlic clove, minced

- 1/2 cup canned tomatoes

- ¼ cup fresh basil leaves, roughly chopped
- 1/4 teaspoon chili powder 1/2 tablespoon olive oil

- 2 whole eggs

- Pepper to taste

How To:

1.   Preheat your oven to 375 degrees F.

2.   Take alittle baking dish and grease with vegetable oil .
3.   Add garlic, basil, tomatoes chili, vegetable oil into a dish and stir.

4.   Crack eggs into a dish, keeping space between the 2 .
5.   Sprinkle the entire dish with sunflower seeds and pepper.

6.   Place in oven and cook for 12 minutes until eggs are set and tomatoes are bubbling.

7.   Serve with basil on top.

Enjoy!

Nutrition (Per Serving)

Calories: 235

Fat: 16g

Carbohydrates: 7g

Protein: 14g

Cool Mushroom Munchies

Serving: 2

Prep Time: 5 minute

Cook Time: 10 minutes

Ingredients:

- 4 Portobello mushroom caps
- 3 tablespoons coconut aminos
- 2 tablespoons sesame oil
- 1 tablespoon fresh ginger, minced
- 1 small garlic clove, minced

How To:

1.   Set your broiler to low, keeping the rack 6 inches from the heating source.

2.   Wash mushrooms under cold water and transfer them to a baking sheet (top side down).
3.   Take a bowl and blend in vegetable oil , garlic, coconut aminos, ginger and pour the mixture over the mushrooms tops .
4.   Cook for 10 minutes.
5.   Serve and enjoy!

Nutrition (Per Serving)

Calories: 196

Fat: 14g

Carbohydrates: 14g

Protein: 7g

Banana and Buckwheat Porridge

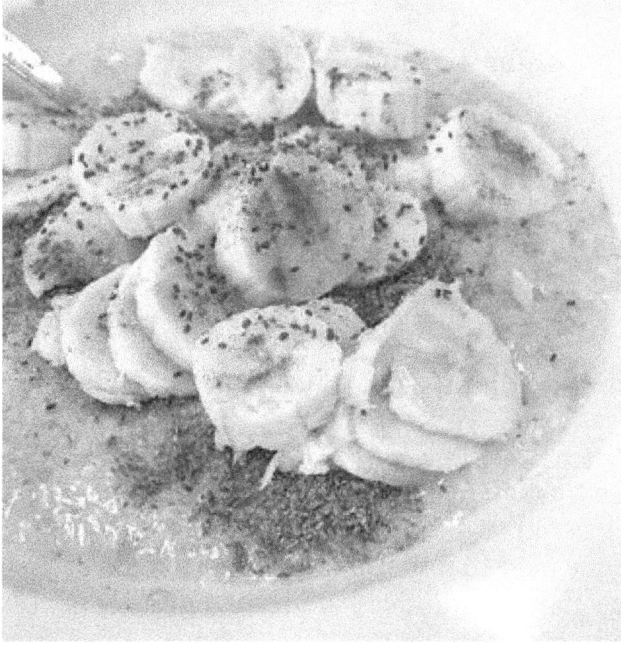

Serving: 2

Prep Time: 10 minutes

Cook Time: 15 minutes

Ingredients:

- 1 cup of water

- 1 cup buckwheat groats

- 2 big grapefruits, peeled and sliced

- 1 tablespoon ground cinnamon

- 3-4 cups almond milk

- 2 tablespoons natural almond butter

How To:

1.   Take a medium-sized saucepan and add buckwheat and water.

2.   Place the pan over medium heat and convey to a boil.
3.   Keep cooking until the buckwheat absorbs the water.
4.   Reduce heat to low and add almond milk, stir gently.
5.   Add the remainder of the ingredients (except the grapefruits).

6.   Stir and take away from the warmth .
7.   Transfer into cereal bowls and add grapefruit chunks.
8.   Serve and enjoy!

Nutrition (Per Serving)

Calories: 223

Fat: 4g

Carbohydrates: 4g

Protein: 7g

Delightful Berry Quinoa Bowl

Serving: 4

Prep Time: 5 minutes

Cook Time: 15 minutes

Ingredients:

- 1 cup quinoa

- 2 cups of water

- 1 piece, 2-inch sized cinnamon stick

- 2-3 tablespoons of maple syrup

- Flavorful Toppings

- ½ cup blueberries, raspberries or strawberries

- 2 tablespoons raisins

1 teaspoon lime

¼ teaspoon nutmeg, grated

- 3 tablespoons whipped coconut cream
- 2 tablespoon cashew nuts, chopped

How To:

1.   Take a metal strainer and pass your grain through them to strain them well.

2.   Rinse the grains under cold water thoroughly.
3.   Take a medium-sized saucepan and pour within the water.
4.   Add the strained grains and convey the entire mixture to a boil.

5.   Add cinnamon sticks and canopy the saucepan.
6.   Lower the warmth and let the mixture simmer for quarter-hour to permit the grain to soak up the liquid.
7.   Remove the warmth and plump up the mixture employing a fork.

8.   Add syrup if you would like additional flavor.
9.   Also, if you're looking to form things a touch more interesting, just add any of the abovementioned ingredients.

Nutrition (Per Serving)

Calories: 202

Fat: 5g

Carbohydrates: 35g

Protein: 6g

Protein: 1.4g

Fantastic Bowl of Steel Oats

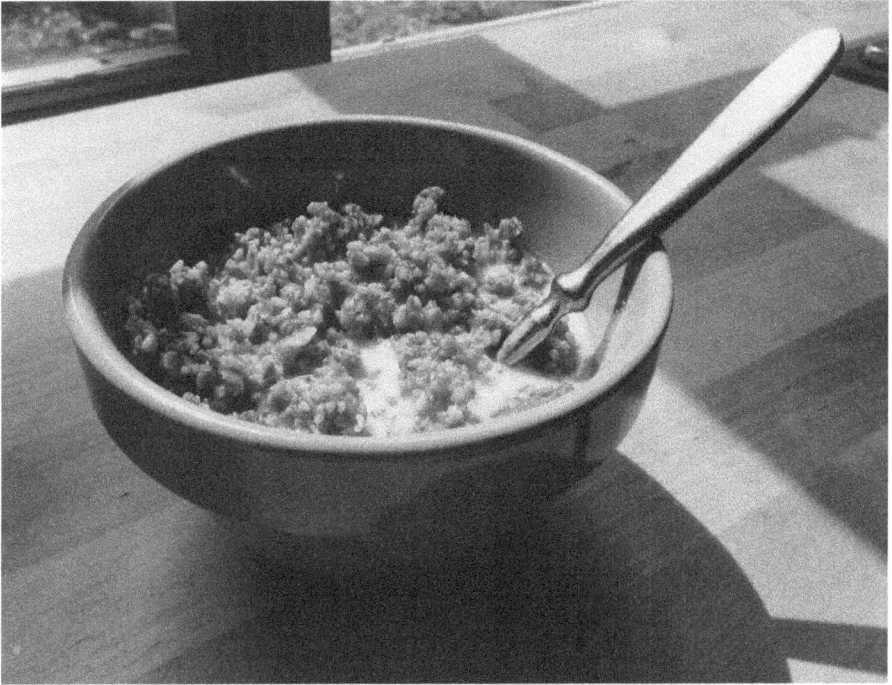

Serving: 4

Prep Time: 5 minutes

Cook Time: 25 minutes

Ingredients:

3 ¾ cup water

1 ¼ cup steel-cut oats

¼ teaspoon salt

Flavorful Toppings

- 1 teaspoon cinnamon

- ½ teaspoon nutmeg

- ½ teaspoon lemon pepper

- 1 teaspoon Garam masala

- Mixed berries as needed

- Diced mangos as needed

- Sliced bananas as needed

- Dried fruits as needed

- Nuts as needed

Flavorful Toppings

- 1 tablespoon coconut milk

How To:

1.   Take a medium-sized saucepan and convey it over high heat.

2.   Add water and permit the water to heat up.

3.   Add the steel-cut oats with some salt and lower the warmth to medium-low.

4.   Let the mixture simmer for about 25 minutes, ensuring to stay stirring it all the way.

5.   Add coconut milk or almond butter for a few extra flavor.

6.   Once done, serve with some berries or nuts.

7.   Enjoy!

Nutrition (Per Serving)

Calories: 125

Fat: 3g

Carbohydrates: 20g

Protein: 7g

Quinoa and Cinnamon Bowl

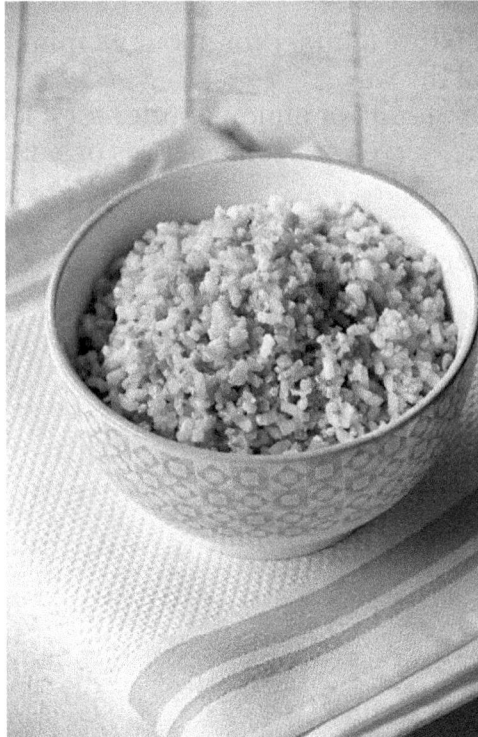

Serving: 2

Prep Time: 10 minutes

Cook Time: 15 minutes

Ingredients:

- 1 cup uncooked quinoa

- 1½ cups water

- ½ teaspoon ground cinnamon

- ½ teaspoon sunflower seeds

- A drizzle of almond/coconut milk for serving

How To:

1.   Rinse quinoa thoroughly underwater.

2.   Take a medium-sized saucepan and add quinoa, water, cinnamon, and seeds.
3.   Stir and place it over medium-high heat.
4.   Bring the combination to a boil.
5.   Reduce heat to low and simmer for 10 minutes.
6.   Once cooked, remove from the warmth and let it cool.
7.   Serve with a drizzle of almond or coconut milk.
8.   Enjoy!

Nutrition (Per Serving)

Calories: 255

Fat: 13g

Carbohydrates: 33g

Protein: 5g

Awesome Breakfast Parfait

Serving: 2

Prep Time: 5 minutes

Cook Time: Nil

Ingredients:

- 1 teaspoon sunflower seeds

- ½ cup low-fat milk

- 1 cup all-purpose flour

- 1 teaspoon vanilla

- 3 eggs, beaten

- 1 teaspoon baking soda

- 2 cups non-fat Greek yogurt

How To:

1.   Hack pretzels into small-sized portions and slice the strawberries.

2.   Add yogurt to rock bottom of the glass and top with pretzel pieces and strawberries.

3.   Add more yogurt and keep repeating until you've got spent all the ingredients.

4.   Enjoy!

Nutrition (Per Serving)

Calorie: 304

Fat: 1g

Carbohydrates: 58g

Protein: 15g

Amazing and Healthy Granola Bowl

Serving: 6

Prep Time: 5 minutes

Cook Time: 25 minutes

Ingredients:

- 1-ounce Porridge oats

- 2 teaspoons maple syrup

- Cooking spray as needed

- 4 medium bananas

- 4 pots of Caramel

- Layered Fromage Frais

- 5 ounce fresh fruit salad, such as strawberries, blueberries, and raspberries

- ¼ ounce pumpkin seeds

- ¼ ounce sunflower seeds

- ¼ ounce dry chia seeds

- ¼ ounce desiccated coconut

How To:

1.   Preheat your oven to 300 degrees F.

2.   Take a baking tray and line with baking paper.
3.   Take an outsized bowl and add oats, syrup , and seeds.
4.   Spread mix on a baking tray.
5.   Spray copra oil on top and bake for 20 minutes, ensuring to stay stirring from time to time.
6.   Sprinkle coconut after the primary quarter-hour .
7.   Remove from oven and let it cool.
8.   Take a bowl and layer sliced bananas on top of the Fromage Fraise.

9.   Spread the cooled granola mix on top and serve with a topping of berries.
10.   Enjoy!

Nutrition (Per Serving)

Calories: 446

Fat: 29g

Carbohydrates: 37g

Protein: 13g

Cinnamon and Pumpkin Porridge Medley

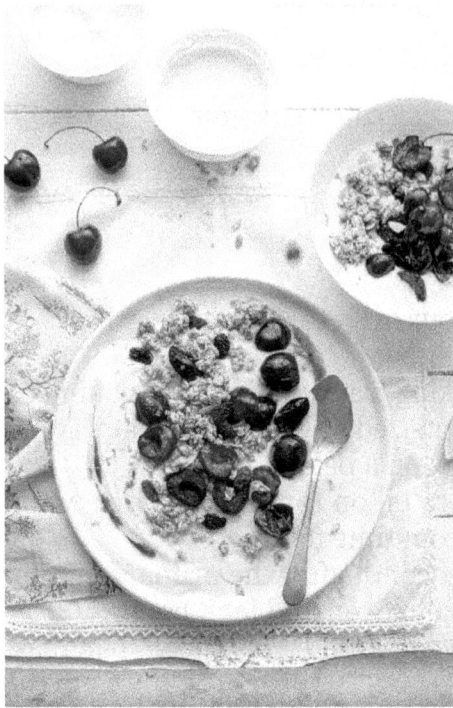

Serving: 2

Prep Time: 10 minutes

Cook Time: 15 minutes

Ingredients:

- 1 cup unsweetened almond/coconut milk

- 1 cup of water

- 1 cup uncooked quinoa

- ½ cup pumpkin puree

- 1 teaspoon ground cinnamon

- 2 tablespoons ground flaxseed meal

- Juice of 1 lemon

How To:

1.   Take a pot and place it over medium-high heat.

2.   Whisk in water, almond milk and convey the combination to a boil.

3.   Stir in quinoa, cinnamon, and pumpkin.
4.   Reduce heat to low and simmer for 10 minutes until the liquid has evaporated.
5.   Remove from the warmth and stir in flaxseed meal.
6.   Transfer porridge to small bowls.
7.   Sprinkle juice and add pumpkin seeds on top.
8.   Serve and enjoy!

Nutrition (Per Serving)

Calories: 245

Fat: 1g

Carbohydrates: 59g

Protein: 4g

Quinoa and Date Bowl

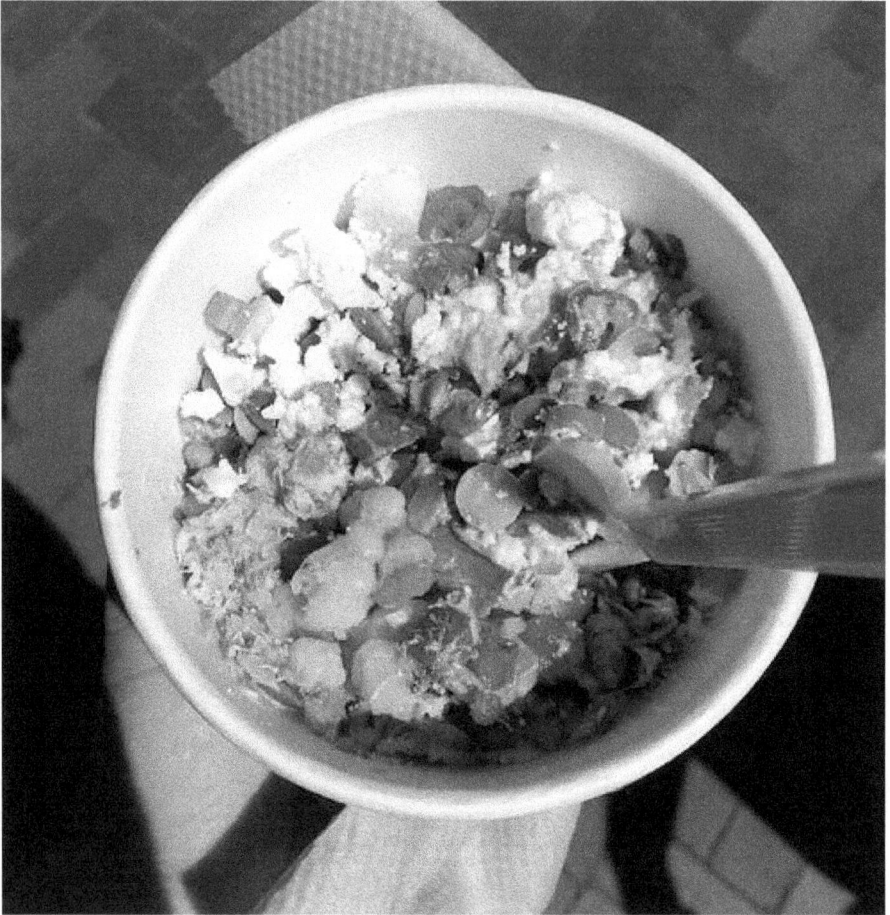

Serving: 2

Prep Time: 10 minutes

Cook Time: 15 minutes

Ingredients:

- 1 date, pitted and chopped finely

- ½ cup red quinoa, dried

- 1 cup unsweetened almond milk

- 1/8 teaspoon vanilla extract

- ¼ cup fresh strawberries, hulled and sliced
- 1/8 teaspoon ground cinnamon

How To:

1. Take a pan and place it over low heat.

2. Add quinoa, almond milk, cinnamon, vanilla, and cook for about quarter-hour , ensuring to stay stirring from time to time.

3. Garnish with strawberries and enjoy!

Nutrition (Per Serving)

Calories: 195

Fat: 4.4g

Carbohydrates: 32g

Protein: 7g

Crispy Tofu

Serving: 8

Prep Time: 5 minutes

Cook Time: 20-30 minutes

Ingredients:

1 pound extra-firm tofu, drained and sliced

- 2 tablespoons olive oil

- 1 cup almond meal

- 1 tablespoons yeast

- ½ teaspoon onion powder ½ teaspoon garlic powder
- ½ teaspoon oregano

How To:

1.   Add all ingredients except tofu and vegetable oil during a shallow bowl.

2.   Mix well.
3.   Preheat your oven to 400 degrees F.
4.   during a wide bowl, add the almond meal and blend well.
5.   Brush tofu with vegetable oil , read the combination and coat well.

6.	Line a baking sheet with parchment paper.
7.	Transfer coated tofu to the baking sheet.
8.	Bake for 20-30 minutes, ensuring to flip once until golden brown.

9.	Serve and enjoy!

Nutrition (Per Serving)

Calories: 282

Fat: 20g

Carbohydrates: 9g

Protein: 12g

Hearty Pumpkin Oats

Serving: 3

Prep Time: 5 minutes

Cook Time: 8 minutes

Ingredients:

- 1 cup quick-cooking rolled oats

- ¾ cup almond milk

- ½ cup canned pumpkin puree

- ¼ teaspoon pumpkin pie spice

- 1 teaspoon ground cinnamon

How To:

1.   Take a secure microwave bowl and add oats, almond milk, and microwave on high for 1-2 minutes.

2.   Add more almond milk if needed to realize your required consistency.
3.   Cook for 30 seconds more.
4.   Stir in pumpkin puree, pie spice, ground cinnamon.
5.   Heat gently and enjoy!

Nutrition (Per Serving)

Calories: 229

Fat: 4g

Carbohydrates: 38g

Protein:10g

Wholesome Pumpkin Pie Oatmeal

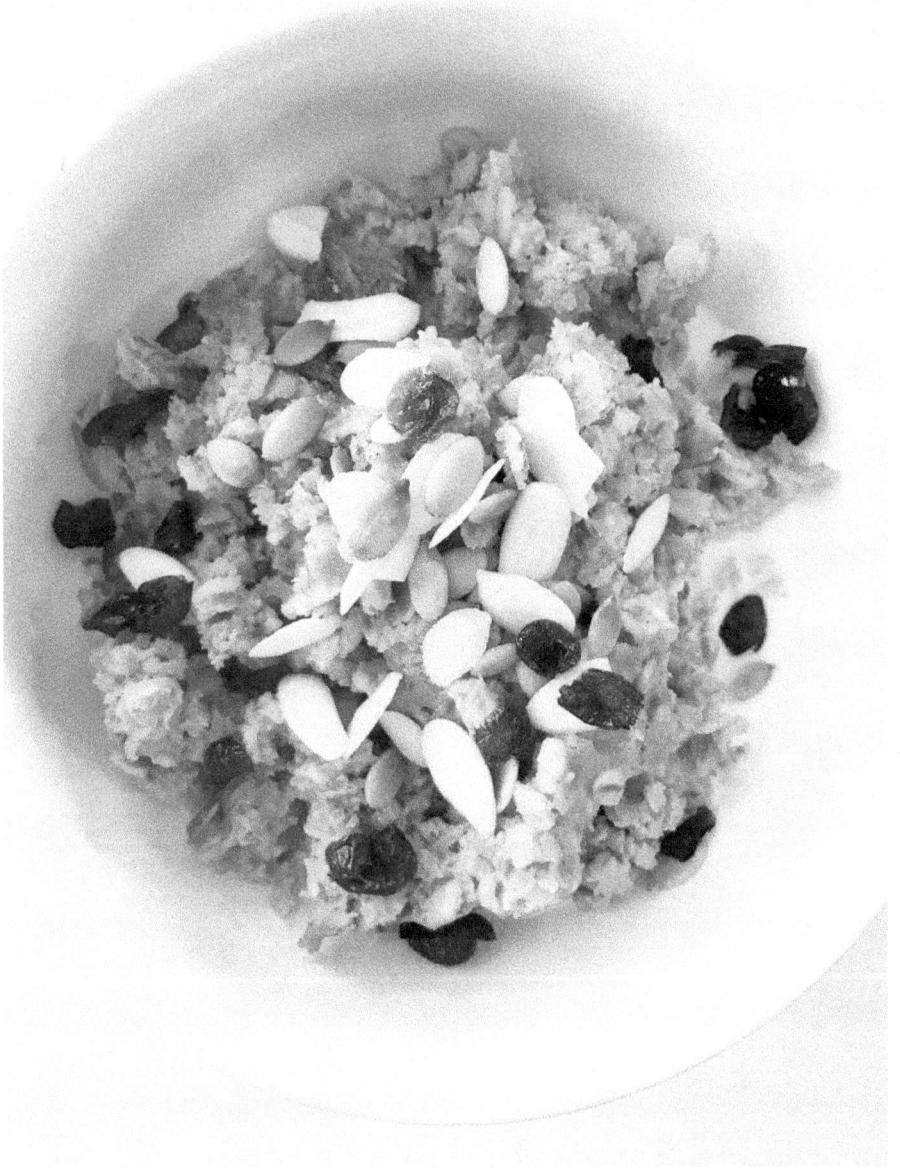

Serving: 2

Prep Time: 10 minutes

Cook Time: 10 minutes

Smart Points: 6

Ingredients:

- ½ cup canned pumpkin, low sodium

- Mashed banana as needed

- ¾ cup unsweetened almond milk

- ½ teaspoon pumpkin pie spice

- 1 cup oats

How To:

1.   Mash banana employing a fork and blend within the remaining ingredients (except oats) and blend well.

2.   Add oats and finely stir.
3.   Transfer mixture to a pot and let the oats cook until it's absorbed the liquid and is tender.
4.   Serve and enjoy!

Nutrition (Per Serving)

Calories: 264

Fat: 4g

Carbohydrates: 52g

Protein: 7g

Power-Packed Oatmeal

Serving: 2

Prep Time: 10-15 minutes

Cook Time: 5 minutes

Ingredients:

- ¼ cup quick-cooking oats

- ¼ cup almond milk

- 2 tablespoons low fat Greek yogurt

- ¼ banana, mashed

- 2-1/4 tablespoons flaxseed meal

How To:

1.   Whisk altogether of the ingredients during a bowl.

2.   Transfer the bowl to your fridge and let it refrigerate for quarter-hour .
3.   Serve and enjoy!

Nutrition (Per Serving)

Calories:

Fat: 11g

Carbohydrates: 27g

Protein: 10g

Chia Porridge

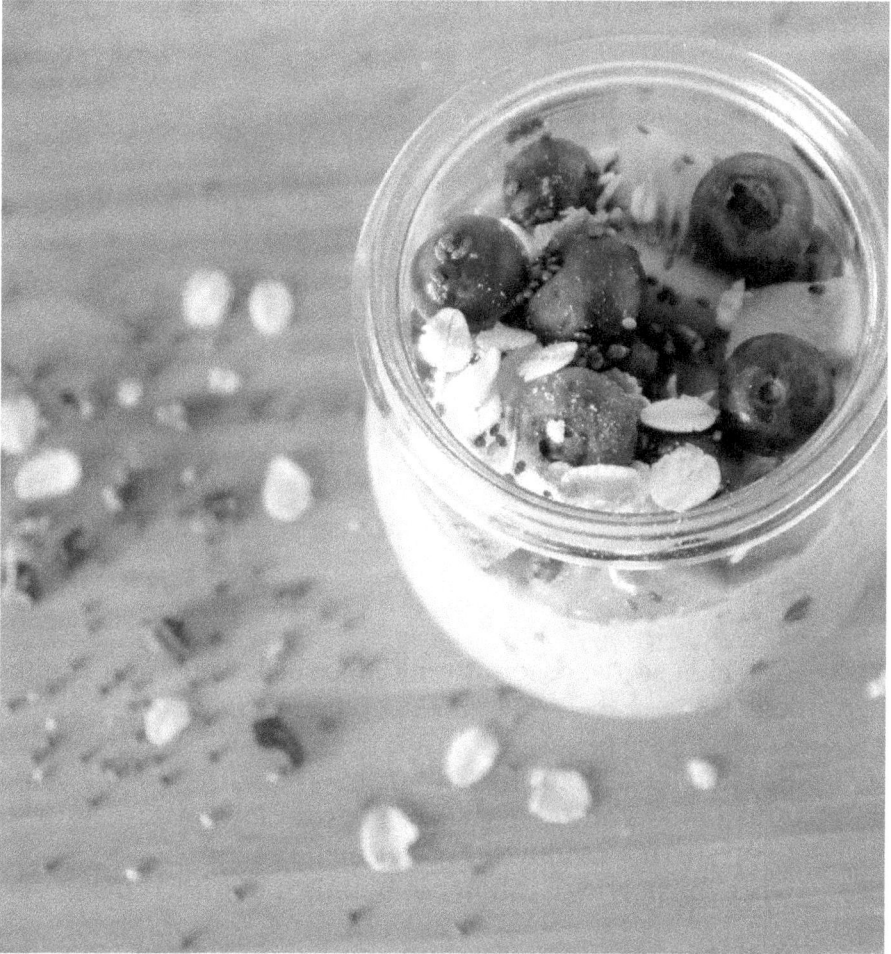

Serving: 2

Prep Time: 10 minutes

Cook Time: 5-10 minutes

Ingredients:

- 1 tablespoon chia seeds

- 1 tablespoon ground flaxseed

- 1/3 cup coconut cream

- ½ cup water

- 1 teaspoon vanilla extract

- 1 tablespoon almond butter

How To:

1.   Add chia seeds, coconut milk , flaxseed, water and vanilla to alittle pot.

2.   Stir and let it sit for five minutes.
3.   Add almond butter and place pot over low heat.
4.   Keep stirring as almond butter melts.
5.   Once the porridge is hot/not boiling, pour into bowl.

6.   Enjoy!

7.   Add a couple of berries or a touch of cream for extra flavor.

Nutrition (Per Serving)

Calories: 410

Fat: 38g

Carbohydrates: 10g

Protein: 6g

www.ingramcontent.com/pod-product-compliance
Lightning Source LLC
Chambersburg PA
CBHW050748030426
42336CB00012B/1711